"Failure Is Not An Option"

Bob & Beverly.
Thankyou for your.
friendship and
support.

Linda

To order additional copies, please contact us.
BookSurge, LLC
www.booksurge.com
1-866-308-6235
orders@booksurge.com

LINDA D'ANGELO

"FAILURE IS NOT AN OPTION"

THRIVING WITH RHEUMATOID ARTHRITIS

2005

"Failure Is Not An Option"

TABLE OF CONTENTS

ACKNOWLEDGEMENTS

To my daughter Samantha
thank you for your love, patience and friendship thank you for
providing me with the courage to go on

To my husband Dave whom I adore,
thank you for your love, understanding and support
thank you for being that special someone whom I can always
count on

The Arthritis Society
thank you for the opportunity to contribute to a select group
of people whom I have something in common with

Family & Friends
thank you for your thoughtfulness, encouragement and
presence in my life

A Special Thank You
special thanks to Schering Canada, Beth Kidd and
Randal F. Allcock at The Village Studio
for their support in the development of my book

To My Daughter Samantha

As you grow into the successful woman I know you will become life will present you with many challenges. These challenges can sometimes be unexpected, undeserved and beyond your control.

It is important to remember that life is never about the challenge itself, it is about you, and how you choose to handle the challenge. Your personal growth, knowledge and learning's come from having the strength of character to step up, face your fears and ascertain your desired outcome.

Through my journey with arthritis we have both come to learn that this illness affects not just the person whom is diagnosed but everyone they are close to. Our journey together has been a long one with many tough times and lots of unknowns. Your love, patience, support and friendship provide me with the courage to go on.

The dedication of this book allows me to continue to express my gratitude and appreciation for the many times you have looked after me when I should have been looking after you.

A daughter truly is a gift from god and I sincerely thank you Samantha for the privilege of mothering you.

FOREWARD
By
Denis Morrice, President
The Arthritis Society of Canada

I f you or a loved one has Rheumatoid Arthritis this book is for you! Linda tells it like it is through her personal journey from diagnosis to now living with regular infusions of Remicade in order to get on with her life.

Linda D'Angelo describes every emotion that one goes through after being diagnosed with rheumatoid arthritis. Prior to her diagnosis there she was a beautiful, determined, confident, successful career woman where any problem in life was simply a challenge to overcome. Linda would overcome each and every challenge life presented her with a smile of victory. Linda's "can do" attitude made her a successful woman. Then at age thirty rheumatoid arthritis hit.

Linda describes the trauma she went through after being diagnosed with what she thought was some 'old persons' disease. One can not help but visualize this incredible young woman sitting on top of the world and then watching it all come tumbling down. A disease like rheumatoid arthritis does not just attack the body, a major side effect is the impact it has on one's energy and self-confidence. Rheumatoid arthritis injects fear of the unknown, despair and sense of no control over one's life.

Once Linda realized that her diagnosis was a life long journey and rheumatoid arthritis would be something she would have to drag along with her the rest of her life she dug deep for her inner strength. She was not going to let the fatigue, pain and negative psychological bullets allow her to become a victim.

I have had the pleasure of knowing Linda for over six years. She is an amazing, courageous woman who has taken the time to share her experience and wisdom with those suffering and affected by this disease. Linda's book will benefit anyone associated with rheumatoid arthritis. I wish her every success with her latest venture "Failure Is Not An Option, Thriving With Rheumatoid Arthritis"

CHAPTER ONE
Leap Of Faith

Today is April 5, 2003, a day to celebrate. The Government of Alberta has finally approved the use of the biologic drugs Remicade and Enbrel, for people suffering from rheumatoid arthritis (RA). I feel so lucky; it is hard to believe that two and half years ago my arthritis was out of control. The deformity in my joints was well underway and pain and fatigue were a constant way of life for me. To make matters worse, I was on the path to realizing my worst nightmare, a wheelchair.

When I started taking Remicade on December 7, 2000, my daughter Samantha was 12 years old. As a single mother who had struggled with RA over the previous eight years, no one was more aware than I was that I needed a miracle and I was hoping that Remicade would be my wonder drug. As my health continued to deteriorate I worried that if this drug did not work, like all of the others I had tried in the past, there was a very real possibility that life for me was going to deteriorate. I found this prospect frightening.

I was going to bed exhausted and waking up in terrible pain. I was always tired and my mobility was becoming a real issue. I was having difficulty walking up and down the twelve steps in my home. House cleaning, laundry and going out to do simple tasks like grocery shopping, banking and other errands were a major chore. Life was becoming more structured every passing day and it scared me to death.

Before my rheumatologist, Dr. Christopher Penny, prescribed Remicade I felt like a sick old woman in a young person's body. I felt defeated and robbed of my life. Knowing that my RA would only get worse was an even tougher pill to swallow. I had to continue to believe that no matter what the future had in store for me "failure was not an option." This mantra became my personal motto. I decided when I was first diagnosed with RA in November 1992 that under no circumstances would I surrender to this illness. I had to be in command of my arthritis and not let it control me. There was, and continues to be, too much at stake and this is one battle I must win. I have to beat this terrible illness, end of story.

The cost of new biologic treatments like Remicade and Enbrel are very expensive, approximately $17,000 - $20,000 per year per patient. Remicade costs about $1,000 per vial and it is prescribed based on body weight. At 130 pounds I need three of these vials, which adds up to $3,000 every eight weeks. I did not know anyone at the time, or today for that matter, who has that kind of disposable income. I had tried every RA drug on the market as well as alternative therapies and medicines claiming to have positive effects for people suffering from RA with little to no success. Therefore, I was ecstatic to be invited to join the trial program sponsored by Schering Canada, the pharmaceutical company that manufactures Remicade. Schering sponsored this program until the federal government approved Remicade and Enbrel for use in Canada in October 2000.

To the surprise of the patients in the trial program, we learned that each province must apply individually to have these biologic drugs added to their drug benefit formulary. Even though the federal government approved Remicade and Enbrel for use, it did not mean that people suffering from RA across the country would have access to them. As a group of patients who were now experiencing an improved quality of life, we were concerned about our future. We were aware that adding a new medication to a provincial formulary could take anywhere from one to four years. With more than 400,000 people in Alberta suffering from arthritis we assumed Alberta would be one of the first provinces to grant access to the new biologic drugs. To our dismay, Alberta was one of the last provinces to add these drugs to its formulary. This left patients like me confused and concerned about whether we would be forced to pay for our expensive medication. For over a year and a half I showed up every eight weeks at the Rockyview Hospital unsure if I would receive my Remicade treatment. And should I be lucky enough to be given my Remicade, I prayed to God that someone else would pay for it.

The panic I and so many others experienced during this time was maddening. There were about 230 Albertans on this trial program. We were all candidates for either short-term or long-term disability if we didn't receive our medication. With Remicade, those of us with careers were no longer fearful of losing our jobs and livelihoods. We could continue to contribute to the economy and support our families. There were others who had been on short-term and long-term disability who were once again employable (either part-time or full-time) as a result of their medication. For the first time since we were diagnosed with RA, a large number of us felt healthy and were enjoying a better quality of life. If you took a close look at these statistics and built an economic model or business case, it would be evident the cost of approving these biologic drugs in all provinces, especially Alberta, was nominal and would pay for itself in short order. Which begged the question, if it makes sense then why wasn't the Government of Alberta approving these drugs for use?

At this point, it become obvious to me that people suffering from arthritis needed to take action. Like AIDS or cancer patients, we need to advocate on behalf of our illness to generate public awareness and to ensure that anyone suffering from rheumatoid arthritis receives proper medical treatment. Working through the Alberta Arthritis Society, a provincial campaign was designed to target government and key public policy decision makers. The outcome of this initiative included both Remicade and Enbrel being approved and added to the provincial formulary for use by Albertans. Much like the illness itself, the approval process for both these drugs was uncertain, chronic and painful for so many people, like me, who so desperately need Remicade and/or Enbrel to maintain their quality of life.

It has been two and half years and Remicade has made a huge difference in my life. It was indeed the wonder drug and miracle I was so desperately searching for. Remicade is not a cure for RA and I am unsure how long I will continue to feel healthy. Remember, this is a new medication with no proven track record, but right now life is incredibly good and I am going to enjoy it. I feel great and I am in excellent health. For now it would appear that my RA has gone into remission and I have my life back.

I recall the anxiety that accompanied my first Remicade treatment. I woke up tired and in pain with 24 swollen joints, I prayed for a miracle. Over the previous two months I started experiencing RA in my hip, which was new and knocked me out of commission for a week every time it would flare up. Having never experienced RA in my hip, I did not have the coping mechanisms in place to deal with the pain. I was feeling powerless, scared and very vulnerable. This illness was silently, and without warning, claiming and destroying all my joints. Remicade was billed as the latest and greatest in RA medications and having tried every drug on the market it was apparent to me that this new medication had to work or my RA was going to cripple me.

I started my Remicade treatment with two other patients; one who moved and I lost touch with, and the other who I now consider a friend. Unfortunately, they both left the program due to complications with their treatment. I was left as the only participant in our initial group. The young lady I met was named Darlene; she was in her 30s with severe deformity in her hands and wrists with a number of fused joints. Her mobility was extremely limited and she showed up for her first treatment using a walker. Each treatment was three to four hours long so through our conversations I came to learn that she lived alone and held down a job pumping gas at a service station. I was astonished that anyone in her condition could do such a job. Her fingers and hands were severely disfigured and deformed due to the progression of her RA.

The gentlemen I met and consider my friend, was named Clem. He was in his 50s and was confined to a wheelchair with a number of deformed joints. He had been cut down in the prime of his life by RA and was no longer able to work. Seeing Clem would trigger thoughts of me realizing my own worst fear, me seated in a wheelchair. However, what really struck me about Clem was his bravery and courage to live life to the fullest. Clem had a great sense of humor and an enthusiasm for life that most healthy people seem to lack. Considering we were all in pain and experiencing a myriad of emotions from hope to fear, Clem was very calm and reassuring. Around Clem, you just didn't think about all the "what ifs" and "could bes" that plagued you throughout the life of this illness. I knew the moment I met Clem that he was one of those special people who exists to inspire us all.

Well wonder drug it turned out to be! After one infusion, Clem left his wheelchair behind and started sporting a walker. Darlene left her walker behind for a cane and I felt like I could run the next marathon. Within 48 hours several of my RA symptoms started to vanish. I woke up refreshed with just moderate pain and had energy to burn at the end of the day. When I arrived for my second Remicade treatment I had 12 swollen joints and moderate pain. By my third treatment, I progressed to 6 swollen joints with minimal pain. This was truly a miracle; it was the wonder drug I was so desperately searching for and needed.

The phenomenon of feeling well led to longer days with more physical activity and socializing. I found myself becoming less rigid with my living habits and schedule than I had been in the past. If my daughter Samantha had something going on we definitely both made it there. If there was a television show I wanted to watch, I stayed up that extra hour. If there was something I wanted to do, I simply did it. When symptoms of my RA would re-appear it was usually because I had over indulged in an old habit I had long-ago abandoned or a new experience I normally would not have engaged in. It was odd because my RA had always meant pain and fatigue to me. Now, I had to remind myself that just because I was feeling healthy and living well, I still had arthritis. With the success of Remicade it became apparent that with a healthy life style, plenty of rest, a proper diet and stress management that I would thrive in spite of this illness.

Remicade has given me my life back and I owe a huge debt of thanks to my rheumatologist, Christopher Penny, who recommended me for this treatment and to Schering Canada for sponsoring me into this program. Today I no longer worry about whether I will be able to care for Samantha. To borrow the old Nike slogan, I just do it. With my family living in Toronto there was always the fear and concern over who will look after Samantha if I can't. Back-up systems need to be put in place when you are single mom who is ill and your family lives half-way across the country. These days I am feeling healthy and living with less stress. My daughter is doing great as a person and we are doing great as a family of two. I feel optimistic and in control of my illness. We have started traveling quite a bit together and are able to have some great outings that we previously would never have embarked upon. I can also keep up with Samantha in the mall and venture there on my own more often. I am enjoying shopping again; it is not the chore it once was for me.

With my health back we are making great memories and sharing a number of meaningful moments and life experiences together. We have been house boating, sea-doing, camping, hiking and enjoying the mountains and great outdoors that Alberta has to offer. We have traveled to Disney World a number of times, have been on a few cruises and this summer I am taking Samantha to New York City to celebrate her Grade Nine graduation. I am very proud of her and excited that we can take this trip to NYC together. This will be one more life experience with mom she can add to her travel album that would not have been possible in the past.

My relationship with my fiancé, soon to be husband, is great. Dave is a wonderful man, who, in the short time I have known him, has been very supportive of my illness and me as a person. Many men say, "don't worry honey, everything will be fine" and some of those same men commit to you "for better or worse" but then are nowhere to be found when you really need them. I have come to learn that it takes a special person to stand by you through something as devastating as RA and Dave has proven he is one of the few special people in this world who are up to the challenge. Being with someone who has a chronic illness is not for the faint of heart.

Dave has cut short or cancelled many business trips to help me when my RA was out of control and I could not care for myself or Samantha. He has seen it all with me and this terrible illness. What constantly amazes me, and what I have grown to appreciate and take comfort in, is that despite the good, bad or the ugly he continues to show up. I feel blessed to have such a strong, loving, caring man beside me who I know will always make things OK and will be at my side for better or worse. Over the last two and half years we have traveled to many places together including Thailand, Malaysia, Mongolia and China. I am learning how to ski so I can venture out on the slopes with Dave on occasion. Together we have taken a few ski weekends in Panorama, B.C., which I never would have dreamed possible, and they have been so much fun. With my RA in remission I am looking forward to experiencing so much more together.

Family and friends are an important part of life, as RA impacts not just you but everyone close to you. The chronic pain and fatigue associated with this illness does not lend itself to a carefree, spontaneous way of life. With both family obligations and social commitments there are days when you have nothing left to give anyone else, because you are struggling just to get by. Therefore, it is important that you surround yourself with family and friends who understand your illness, how it affects you and how you deal with it. I consider myself fortunate to have such wonderful family and friends who have been loyal, compassionate, supportive and understanding of me, my illness, my contribution to The Arthritis Society and my quest to conquer RA.

Career-wise, I am at the top of my game and I am having a lot of fun. My colleagues are aware of my RA and are supportive, understanding and caring. I have taken on a number of new assignments that took me out of my normal routine and allowed me to travel. It is making life a little more interesting. I am also participating in a number of industry associations in a significant way and that reflects well on my company as well as adds to my personal and professional development and growth. I feel happy and challenged.

Five years ago I contacted Cathy Miller, the Alberta and Northwest Division Executive Director for The Arthritis Society. I told her I wanted to understand more about my illness and that it was time for me start to contribute to an organization and a group of people with whom I have something in common. I want to make a difference and improve the quality of life for people like me, who suffer from arthritis. During this period I have become knowledgeable about arthritis-related issues and I have had the pleasure of meeting some of the most wonderful people in the most adverse circumstances. I derive a lot of pleasure and satisfaction from my volunteer work with The Arthritis Society as it provides me the opportunity to contribute and make a difference.

Personally, I have passed some major milestones. I have come to accept that I have this terrible illness and I have had to re-invent and re-create a life that works for me, since the life I knew before my diagnosis was not going to carry me into the future. With no cure for RA on the horizon, my future will remain uncertain. Having said that, today it appears that my RA has gone into remission so I am going seize the opportunity and enjoy life.

I treasure and value my relationships with my daughter, my fiancé, my family and my friends. My career is important to me; it is not only my livelihood but it provides the personal and professional growth and development I crave. My dedication to The Arthritis Society allows me to contribute to a select group of people with whom I have something in common. My personal accomplishments are many, including learning to ski, climbing the Great Wall of China and riding a camel through the Gobi Desert. I am a young woman with a bright future in front of me and I want to experience all that life has to offer. I am going to beat this illness. Experience has taught me that with the right attitude you too can realize your dreams and thrive with RA.

Whether you are newly diagnosed with this illness, or a RA veteran wondering whether you will ever experience a normal life again, my advice to you is fight and fight hard. Your quality of life and the lives of all those close to you are at risk. Like you, I have traveled this painful journey, afraid, confused, alone and terrified about the future. With no cure in sight, I know my journey has not come to an end and I may be travelling that hard road once again.

Through this experience I have come to learn that life presents you with a number of challenges so you need to consider your RA a challenge. These challenges can sometimes be unexpected, undeserved and beyond your control. Therefore, it is important to remember that life is never about the challenge itself, it is about you and how you choose to face the challenge.

Your personal growth, knowledge and learning's come from the strength of character to step up, face your fears and ascertain your desired outcome, thriving with RA. If you want quality of life for you and those close to you, failure is not an option!

CHAPTER TWO
Diagnosis

I was 30 years old when I was first diagnosed with Rheumatoid Arthritis (RA) in 1992. I remember sitting in the office of my rheumatologist, Dr. Gilbert Fagnou, on a dreary November day eager to find out what was wrong with me. After months of pain, numerous visits to my family physician and internal medicine specialists and the myriad of tests I had undergone at the hospital over the last two months, this "thing" that was wrong with me would finally get a name. While waiting for Dr. Fagnou to return with my results I thought to myself: Life these last four months has been hard and what a relief it will be to finally discover what is wrong with me so I can start dealing with it. I need to get on with my life!

My thoughts were interrupted with the news that I had been diagnosed with rheumatoid arthritis, (RA). I looked at my rheumatologist in disbelief and asked him if he had made a mistake or maybe got my test results mixed up with someone else's records. Arthritis was "an old person's illness" and I was not an old person. I was 30 years old with a 3 year old daughter, in the prime of my life. Again my thoughts were interrupted when he told me there are more than 100 forms of arthritis with rheumatoid, osteoarthritis, gout and lupus being the most common.

My rheumatologist continued with a candid and more

detailed explanation about RA and how it may or may not affect me. I learned that RA was more prominent in women than men. One in seven women over the age of 25 will be diagnosed with RA and the prevalence rates are higher in women after child birth. RA primarily affects the synovial joints of the body and usually attacks many joints simultaneously. RA typically attacks the same joints on both sides of the body with the dominant side often more severely affected. Joint stiffness, pain and swelling, accompanied by fatigue, are typical symptoms experienced by RA patients. Pain is caused by inflamed cells and chemicals that affect the nerve endings within the joints. The thin synovial membrane becomes inflamed and then activates and releases enzymes and chemicals that permanently damage the cartilage and the bone. These enzymes and chemicals also attract more cells into the inflamed tissue. The inflammation caused by RA can lead to joint destruction and deformity.

In a very matter of fact tone, with little bedside manner, my rheumatologist informed me that if my RA was not properly treated I would become crippled. It would mean giving up my career and future earning power, losing my spouse, family and friends. What hit me the hardest is that people diagnosed with RA die at a younger age than the general population. He said if I did not receive early and proper treatment my future would look very different than what I had envisioned for myself. I felt overwhelmed and on the verge of tears. Along with the knowledge that my life was going to change forever, my rheumatologist presented me with a prescription, a follow up appointment, a few pamphlets explaining RA and a contact number for The Arthritis Society.

I left his office in a fog, suddenly realizing this is more than just pain in my hands and feet. Life for me was going to change dramatically. I felt vulnerable, afraid, confused and terrified about the future. I remember thinking now was not the time to panic. I needed to find the strength and courage to remain calm and deal with this.

I stopped at a café in the lobby of the building and ordered a coffee. I needed some time to process all this information before I picked up Samantha from the babysitter and told my husband Stew of my diagnosis. My hands and feet were inflamed and throbbing; it was only a matter of time before my head would be feeling the same way. The heat from the cup of coffee comforted my hands for a few moments and interrupted the myriad of passing thoughts. My mind was racing. Perhaps I'm in shock, I thought, staring into my coffee. Life is good. I have a happy marriage, a great daughter and a fulfilling career. I am doing all the things that I want to do. So why me? Why now?

I remember thinking: Clearly this illness is going to affect not just me but everyone close to me. As the primary caregiver in our household it became apparent that I was going to require assistance and support adjusting to this illness. With my family living in Toronto and my husband attached to a military operational unit and away most of the time, what was help going to look like for me? I played a number of different scenarios over in my mind and none seemed practical or made any sense. I had always been independent. I had lived abroad for many years and moved from province to province within Canada. For the first time in my life the reality of being alone set in and it was unsettling. Unaware of how much time had passed and void of any answers to my questions I decided to leave the café and head home.

After I put Samantha to bed I sat down with Stew and explained what I had learned that afternoon. Stew said all the right things and reassured me that "everything was going to be fine." This was new territory for the both of us, as neither of us had been seriously ill or required long-term support before. Based on our history together I was the strong one who took care of things and made things happen since Stew spent so much time away from home. In all honesty, Stew's laid back reaction to the news of my illness caused me concern. I wondered whether Stew had it in him to step up and take care of me when he was so used to me taking care of him. I also questioned whether our relationship would suffer and fall apart like so many others my rheumatologist told me about? Or would our relationship have the strength to weather my illness. Tired from the events of the day and confused about so many things I went to bed secure in the knowledge that this would all be here for me to deal with in the morning. Tomorrow is another day and after a good night's rest, life may look a little brighter.

The following day, my closest girlfriend Ritu called me to ask about the results of my rheumatologist's appointment. When I told her the diagnosis she rushed right over to my home and we had a long chat about my illness and how I was coping with all of this. It felt good to speak openly about matters that were weighing heavily on my mind. Ritu has always been very supportive no matter what the situation and I knew that I could count on her to be there for me. Shortly after my diagnosis, Ritu moved to Kingston, Ontario then Jacksonville, Florida. Even from a distance she continues to be a loyal friend. We both know that the lines of communication are always open and we visit each other when our schedules allow. Having said that, I really miss not having her here in Calgary and living close by.

I also called my parents in Toronto and let them know

about my diagnosis. Much like me, they were surprised to find out I had been diagnosed with RA, especially since there was no previous history of any form of arthritis within our family. They were concerned that the distance would not allow them to be there for me the way they would have liked too. However, we are a close family and speak to each other weekly so I knew I could always count on them for morale support.

After reviewing the pamphlets my rheumatologist gave me I was armed with the knowledge that RA does not affect everyone in the same way. Just as people have different personalities, arthritis has different temperaments. These temperaments are known as mild, moderate and severe. In most patients, the type of temperament diagnosed at the onset persists during the entire course of the disease. Thirty per cent of patients are diagnosed with mild RA. In some patients the disease may run a short course but in others it recurs intermittently or is constantly present for years. Damage or deformity of joints with mild RA is uncommon. Thirty to forty per cent of patients are diagnosed with moderate RA and it often involves the hands, wrists, elbows, knees or feet. If left untreated, moderate RA can lead to joint damage and deformity. Ten per cent of patients are diagnosed with severe RA. In these cases, normal functions are profoundly affected and aggressive treatment is required to control damage to joints and deformity.

I had a number of inflamed and painful joints as well as chronic fatigue and was diagnosed with moderate RA. My illness progressed quickly causing intense pain, further fatigue, joint damage and the onset of deformity in my hands. It became evident I needed the right mix of medications to cope with the day-to-day symptoms of this illness to limit its progression and long-term effects. In so much pain and exhausted a majority of the time, this illness was wearing me down and taking its toll on every day life. I was no longer the independent woman I once knew. I started requiring assistance with many tasks around the house. Simple things like lifting laundry baskets, vacuuming and other housework caused me a lot of pain. I not only wanted someone to lighten the load at home, there were days I needed someone to take care of me.

Over the following two years my arthritis became increasingly severe and the pain and fatigue associated with it were now out of control. Despite the numerous medications I had tried, the pain and fatigue were overwhelming and it was becoming increasingly difficult to manage. Without the right medication, or combination of medications, I could not control this illness and I was no longer the person I knew prior to my diagnosis. I felt like a sick old woman in a young person's body. I felt defeated and robbed of my life. So many of my fears were being realized, I was living in pain, afraid, confused, alone and terrified about what the future had in store for me.

From the very onset of my diagnosis, I found it most disturbing that Stew chose not to inform himself about my illness. As a result, he did not understand the illness itself or its effects. Therefore, Stew could not support me the way I needed him too. During this time he must have said countless times "don't worry honey, everything will be fine." He didn't seem to understand that "everything was not fine" and would never be "fine" for me again or "fine" for us as a family. His lack of support and understanding made me angry and I could feel resentment building inside me. If I was going to beat this illness I needed an equal partner, and we were not equals. He refused to educate himself about the biggest thing that had ever happened to either of us and it became evident that I was on my own in this fight.

Whether it was a coping mechanism or whether I was in denial, a pattern took shape during this period in my life. I was not crying or grieving over my diagnosis with RA and how it was affecting me and our family life. I was also not admitting my fears or speaking to people honestly about my illness, including my girlfriend Ritu or my parents. With both of them far away, communication was a challenge. My RA was progressing faster than I could have anticipated and my health was deteriorating at the same speed. It took time and energy to explain all the details and I opted out. It was just easier not to say anything.

With others who were unaware of my illness, I did not feel the need to inform them. Life was becoming increasingly more challenging and I was struggling with so many activities that at one time seemed so basic. I no longer felt capable of performing the everyday activities I once took for granted and as a result I was losing confidence in myself. I felt too ashamed to acknowledge and inform others that I was ill with RA because I did not want to be perceived as inferior or deemed less of a person. I was no longer myself and I no longer had the ability and energy to live my life the way I had before my diagnosis. Life seemed so damned hard these days.

With the unrelenting pain and fatigue of my RA, I found myself either compensating or passing up opportunities to take part in activities and outings I once enjoyed. I did not look like I had RA, I appeared fine so no one questioned me about the change in my behavior and I did not bother to inform them about the real problem. As far as everyone was concerned, I was happy, healthy and had a great life.

With the progression of my illness, the demands of raising Samantha, running a household and keeping my career afloat were becoming onerous. There were days I was in so much pain I had nothing left to give anyone else. I was physically, emotionally and mentally exhausted, I was just trying to survive. The strong woman I once knew was slowly slipping away and it scared me to death. It became apparent that I was doing too much and I needed to slow down. I was in pain and tired all the time. Continuing at this pace would only cause another flare up and knock me out of commission for a week at a time. More often than not I found myself living in a cocoon of pain, immobile and unable to care for myself. I was not living the life I had envisioned for myself. I merely existed through each passing day. I desperately needed to find the right medication or combination of medications to control the inflammation; otherwise I would not be able to manage this illness.

During the first year and a half of my illness I had several appointments with my rheumatologist. I was treated with numerous first-line drugs referred to as nonsteroidal anti-inflammatory drugs (NSAIDs) as well as a variety of second-line drugs referred to as disease modifying anti-rheumatic drugs (DMARDs). NSAIDs are the first level of therapy for most arthritic diseases; they lower fever, relieve pain and reduce inflammation. There are more than twenty NSAIDs on the market and they are available in many forms. They can be taken orally, as creams or as suppositories. DMARDs are proven to slow the progression of joint damage and deformity caused by RA. These drugs require approximately three to twelve weeks to work effectively. DMARDs are also known to sometimes have significant adverse reactions and require ongoing monitoring by a doctor.

Neither the first-line or second-line medications I was prescribed had much effect or success in suspending the progression of my RA. This list included Celebrex, a new medication that is used to reduce the pain, stiffness and inflammation of RA while protecting patients from gastrointestinal bleeding often caused by traditional NSAIDs. The major advantage of this type of treatment is the reduced frequency of ulcers.

The DMARDs prescribed included methotrexate, which is taken both orally and by injection. This is the therapy of choice for treating moderate to severe RA since it can be taken in combination with other DMARDs. Plaquenil, Sulfasalazine and Minocin were also prescribed to me in combination with other DMARDs for severe RA.

Due to the lack of success, my rheumatologist decided to add Solganol gold treatments to the mix. When gold works, the response is dramatic. Gold is one of the few drugs that can bring about a complete remission that lasts for years. Although I did not experience complete remission, I did realize significant improvement with the pain and inflammation. For a year and a half I enjoyed the benefits of feeling better, life was not great but it was not the grind I had become accustomed too. I went to my general practitioner weekly for gold injections fully aware of the associated side effects. Gold treatments warrant monthly blood testing to monitor kidney damage and protein in the urine. Skin rash is the mildest and most common side effect experienced with gold treatments and can be detected visually.

In addition to the gold treatments, adopting a healthy lifestyle, paying attention to my RA symptoms, reading my body and learning my limitations was paramount. Now more than ever, attention to detail made the difference when it came to energy and how much I had to expend. Proper nutrition, plenty of rest, regular exercise and managing my stress would assist me in my quest to beat this illness. With a positive attitude and healthy lifestyle I felt I could regain some control, influence my quality of life and better care for Samantha.

Through trial and error I learned it is important to set realistic goals for myself and to seek help when required. If there is no aid or support available it is essential that I prioritize what is important and shorten my list of things to do. I have learned that one of the keys to managing this illness is balance and not stressing out over matters I can not control. It is important to let those close to me know my limitations and ask for help when I need it.

I was approaching my third anniversary with RA and for the first time in a long time I was starting to regain some control of my life. I had a general understanding of my illness and was becoming aware of my personal triggers in an effort to reduce the flare-ups. I was persistent and finally found a combination of drugs that provided me with some relief from the pain and inflammation caused by everyday life. With any luck it would also prevent the progression of my illness so I could avoid further joint damage, disfiguration and deformity. Since my body was behaving itself, it became easier and easier for me to pretend that everything was fine. As a result of the many struggles I had experienced over the last three years and the sense of normalcy I so desperately craved for, I had yet to contact The Arthritis Society as instructed by my rheumatologist when I was first diagnosed with RA.

I knew I was ill and everything was not fine, but personally I was not ready to go public with my RA yet. Yes, life was a little easier these days but I was still struggling with the ongoing pain and fatigue that plagued me everyday. I had not conquered or beat this illness yet and I wasn't feeling confident that I could. In this fragile emotional state I did not want to go to meetings, gather with other people suffering from RA and learn about how this illness may or may not affect my future. I was not ready for that yet. I knew I could not cope with meeting someone in the advanced stages of this illness since it would be my worst fear realized.

Instead, I chose to focus on raising Samantha and on my career. At age six Samantha was becoming less physically challenging for me to care for. There was no longer a need for me to carry around those heavy diaper bags loaded with extra changes of clothes, formula and baby food. Samantha was able to bath herself with some supervision and we could eat out easily. All in all, she was maturing into a mobile, self-sufficient youngster. Mothering Samantha was becoming less physically demanding. Samantha was a good-natured and happy child and a pleasure to care for. I enjoyed doing a lot of things with her from outings to just staying home and playing with her toys. Mothering Samantha has made me a better person and has been a real privilege.

During this difficult time in my life the one person I took much delight and comfort in was Samantha. Her warm, beautiful smile, lots of cuddles and unconditional love and acceptance were just what I needed, especially when I was really ill with a flare up. I consider Samantha a gift from God and I am looking forward to the years ahead. I want to continue to foster a close relationship and build a bond with her that only mothers and daughters share. It is important that I am healthy and beat this illness so I can be a good role model as she continues to develop into the successful young woman I know she will become.

In the early years of my illness I was invited to join a geomatics firm and as a result I sold my consulting business. It was an exciting prospect since I had not been exposed to the oil and gas industry within my consulting business. The position of business development manager in this new company would provide me with a challenge. Early in our negotiations I felt it was important to inform my potential employer about my RA as this could become a problem should my illness continue to progress. It was important to me that, prior to accepting this position, the General Manager understood I was a mother first, had an illness I could not control and both would require some flexibility on their part regarding time off. For me, it was only after these two priorities were met that the rest of the world came into play. After what seemed to be a very long discussion about my illness and many questions about how I was managing and coping with it, the offer was still on the table. We shook hands and I started the following week.

Looking back at my four years with Challenger Surveys & Services I experienced an increasing number of flare ups with my RA due to the many demands that go along with working for a growing organization. In an effort to prove my worth, my schedule had become busier than I was accustomed to when working for myself. Overall, life was speeding along at a heightened pace. Working full-time in a management position that included travel was tiring so it was important for me to bring additional structure to my already disciplined lifestyle. A strict diet, exercise and lots of rest would allow me to increase my energy level and reduce stress. Despite the increase in my flare-ups, my medications were working and for the first time in a long time I was feeling better and having fun. During this time I learned a lot about myself and what I was capable of. I had many successes, which restored my personal confidence and my ability to better cope with my RA. My supervisor, Dave, and I had a good relationship and as a result he was very intuitive and seemed to know when I was having a tough time with my RA. When Dave realized I was struggling he would often say "you have been working really hard, why don't you take the afternoon or the day off, you have earned it." Not wanting to admit defeat, I would smile and say "thank you" and head home to get the extra rest I needed to manage the pain and fatigue associated with this illness.

Just when life was starting to look somewhat normal, my gold treatments started to lose their effect. After consulting with my rheumatologist I learned this was not uncommon. My bubble had burst and once again my RA was becoming more severe. I was not fine and there was no point in kidding myself that I would be. Again, I was on the hunt for a new medication or combination of medications that would provide me with some relief. This journey was becoming all too familiar and the time had come to fight for what was important to me, my quality of life.

After an unexpectedly challenging day at the office my fingers, hands and wrists were hot, red and inflamed. Dave noticed this and asked how I was managing. I said I'd had better days. Stressed, tired and in pain, my guard was down and I started to cry. This was the first time I had become emotional in public and I was mortified. I thought to myself, "Girl, what the heck has come over you? What are you doing crying at the office?" Whatever it was, I had to pull myself together and fast, this was not appropriate behavior for the office. Sensing the panic I was experiencing, Dave closed my office door and I informed him about my medication losing its effect and we talked about my fears and the challenges ahead. We talked for a long time and during our discussion I came to realize that I did not need to fight this battle alone. There are resources available to me if I chose to take advantage of them.

This illness is a lot for one person to deal with and frankly, I was tired of feeling afraid, confused, alone and terrified about the future. The time had come for me to accept the fact that I had RA and contact The Arthritis Society for some support. The feelings of shame and insecurity I was experiencing had to stop. This was no longer about what other people may or may not think of me and my illness or how I am managing and coping with it. The focus needed to be on me and doing what was right for me. I needed to take back control. In my quest to conquer this illness, the time had come for me to get some help and to go public.

CHAPTER THREE
Acceptance Is Key

Based on my experience with this illness it became obvious that in order to conquer my rheumatoid arthritis (RA) and regain my quality of life I needed to acknowledge and accept my RA. After three years of pain, conflict and silence I decided that accepting my RA would give me the confidence to speak openly about my illness, its effects and how I am coping with them. More importantly, I needed to complete the grieving process over the loss of the healthy life I no longer possessed. I needed to let go of my fear of being perceived as inferior and regain the confidence needed to seek assistance, knowledge and support from all known sources available to me. Accepting the fact that I have RA will assist me in my fight to triumph over this awful illness.

Looking back, I remember thinking: Today is a new day and today I will admit that I have been diagnosed with a debilitating illness called RA. Today and every day going forward there will be no more conflict and no more secrets, those who need to know I have RA will be told. Today I am going to turn a page in this story and start a new chapter. Today I am going to contact The Arthritis Society.

As soon as I arrived at my office I reached for the telephone book, searched for the number for The Arthritis Society and noted it in my daytimer. I thought to myself that after my early morning meeting this would be my next point of business. I knew once I picked up the telephone and contacted The Arthritis Society my illness would become public, it would be out there for all to be aware of and maybe pass judgement upon. I was nervous yet feeling like a huge weight was about to be lifted off my shoulders. During my meeting I was distracted, I recall hearing a little voice in the back of my mind speaking to me. The voice urged me to press forward with my plans and to make the call I knew I needed to make. My meeting complete, I went back to my office, picked up the telephone and dialed The Arthritis Society.

When greeted by the receptionist I asked for the name of the Executive Director and requested to speak with her. Cathy Miller and I had a brief discussion about my illness and my desire to learn more about it. I also informed her that I wanted to become involved with The Arthritis Society in a significant way and wondered what opportunities were available for me. We scheduled a lunch meeting for the following week to introduce ourselves, discuss my illness and how I might contribute to the organization.

If acceptance is key, then this telephone call was testimony to my determination in dealing with the loss of an old life that would no longer serve me and all the shame and secrets that went with it. At the time, I was unaware that contacting The Arthritis Society was going to transform my life in a way I could have never imagined. That simple telephone call helped me recreate a new life that would have purpose, be fulfilling and carry me into the future.

The week before my meeting with Cathy was business as usual. A few opportunities presented themselves for me to discuss my illness with my colleagues and I took advantage of them. I was concerned, apprehensive and unaware how things would turn out. I thought to myself "Girl, if you are going to go public there is no time like the present to walk your talk." So, moving forward with a leap of faith, I set out on this journey.

The one memory that captures my "coming out" was replacing the water jug at the office. Part of managing your RA involves maintaining a proper diet and drinking lots of water. I went to the coffee station to fill my water bottle and to my dismay realized the jug was nearly empty and would need replacing when I was finished. I was in so much pain I couldn't lift the water jug into the dispenser. My usual coping mechanism was to head back to my office and wait for someone to finish the last of the water and replace the old jug with a new one. Asking someone for help would only prompt too many questions and an explanation I was not prepared to give. But that day I abandoned my old behaviors drained the last of the water, removed the empty jug and asked one of the fellows in the office to replace it for me.

My worst fears realized, I received the weirdest look and a comment I was not expecting, "What's wrong with you? Are you crippled? Can't you do it yourself?" Taken aback, I eventually responded, "Actually, yes I am close to crippled. I have rheumatoid arthritis and am in a world of hurt right now and can barely move. I would really appreciate it if you could lift this heavy jug in to the water dispenser." Somewhat on the defensive and the verge of tears, nothing could have prepared me for what was going to happen next.

This fellow named Kelly, who was better known as the office clown, turned to me and said, "I'm sorry. I didn't know you had rheumatoid arthritis, I thought old people got arthritis. Does it hurt a lot?" I said, "Yes it does, I have had it for three years now and it is not getting any better and I am in a lot of pain all the time." The water jug quickly replaced, we stood at the coffee station and chatted for some time about my RA. Kelly was very understanding, compassionate and sympathetic. His genuine concern took me from feeling somewhat defensive and on the verge of tears to humble. Completely unaware what a tremendous leap of faith I had taken, Kelly left me with my dignity intact and made my first experience in going public a pleasant one. It was an experience I would repeat over and over again in the next few months.

The week passed and my lunch with Cathy was fast approaching. Setting up this meeting was a huge step forward for me and I was experiencing emotions ranging from anxiety to relief and so many more I did not fully understand. Yet strangely enough I was also looking forward to meeting Cathy and exploring this journey I had set out on. Coming to terms with my illness. Once again a familiar thought crossed my mind: It is time to turn this page and move on to the next chapter.

As a child I was brought up with the knowledge that you only have one chance to make a first impression. What immediately struck me when I first met Cathy was that she was very well put together, compassionate and knowledgeable about RA and arthritis in general. She informed me that she had been in her role for fourteen years and, I later learned, was one of the most well respected Executive Directors within The Arthritis Society in Canada.

Once done with pleasantries and our lunch selection, Cathy gently inquired about my RA and how I was dealing with my illness. We talked at great length about my experiences with RA over the previous three years. It quickly became apparent that there was a great deal I did not understand and it was imperative I learn. We also discussed the role of The Arthritis Society nationally and within Alberta. More informed about the organization, I asked Cathy if there was a role for me to play or an opportunity for me to contribute to this group of people with whom I have something in common.

We spent about an hour and half together and had a pleasant lunch. For the first time ever, I had a meaningful conversation with someone who knew about RA and understood what I was living with mentally, emotionally and physically. When we parted company, Cathy said she would contact me shortly once she had reflected on our discussion in more detail and came up with some ideas and opportunities I would enjoy within The Arthritis Society.

On my way back to the office I pondered our lunch and all that we had discussed. I decided I had made the right decision in contacting The Arthritis Society. Only good was going to come of this meeting and I was overdue in the "good" department when it came to my RA. I felt in control of my destiny and that I would somehow beat this illness and regain my quality of life on a more permanent basis.

Lunch behind me, life went on as usual. When I got home that evening I spoke to Stew about my lunch with Cathy, how it had affected me and my hopes for the future. The entire conversation was a disappointment. The only response the discussion prompted from Stew was "That's great, I'm glad you had a nice lunch." Clearly Stew and I had been on different paths for a while and the divide continued to grow. We wanted different things in life, had different interests and could no longer find common ground. I knew Stew loved me but we were becoming strangers with only Samantha in common. Our relationship would have likely continued in this state for some time but the demands of my RA and the realities of living with a chronic illness forced me to end my relationship with Stew. I moved on to what I hoped would be a better life for Samantha and me.

The old wives tale "things happen in threes" was certainly true in my case. In the span of three months I separated from my husband, bought and moved into a new home and started a new job. During the worst time in my life I was offered an excellent opportunity from a client to join his engineering firm. The opportunities for professional growth and development, in addition to being part of the ownership group, were too good to pass up. As much as I enjoyed my role at Challenger Surveys & Services I had recognized my full potential within this organization. It was time to move on to something more challenging and potentially more lucrative. As a single mother providing for her family, the real attraction was more disposable income. More money meant more security and this was suddenly very important.

My arthritis was already out of control and the stress of starting a new life and a new job accelerated the progression of my RA. The increased inflammation meant I was in a lot of pain. I was losing too much weight, I was run down, tired and in a flare up a majority of the time. During the next six months I was once again feeling defeated and robbed of my life. So many of my fears were being realized, I was living my life in pain, afraid, confused, alone and terrified about what the future had in store for me.

What made matters worse, and increased my level of stress, was the knowledge and fear of being the sole provider in my family. I needed to pay the mortgage, pay the bills, put food on the table, and give myself and Samantha a life we could both be proud of. In order to control my stress and manage my RA, the time had come to treat my personal life like a business. I needed to get out of the trenches and stop doing everything myself. It was imperative that I learn how to become a manager on my illness, learn how to direct the show and work with others to help me get the job done.

When starting a new life, a few essentials are required. I called my girlfriend Marilyn who is a realtor and said we needed to find a house for Samantha and me. With that done in short order, I hired contractors to make a few renovations to turn our new house into a home. Furniture was next on my list of things to do and I under-estimated what a huge undertaking furnishing our home would be. Furniture is neither female nor arthritis friendly so I made a few calls and was fortunate to have two close friends, Don and Dave, available when my furniture arrived to assemble it and move it around the house into its proper place.

The move taught me that the best skill to master is goal setting, understanding what is important, what you need to accomplish and then applying your newfound skills to help you get the job done. In the beginning this process can be a lengthy one because it is new and can require significant effort on your part. But if you stay the course and do not go back to your old familiar ways, this process is invaluable. I learned first hand that the key is to challenge yourself and press forward. If you can master the process, life will become more comfortable and generally easier to manage.

With the essentials now complete it was time to look longer term, what assistance did I require to make life simpler? My home had to be arthritis friendly and well planned to avoid extra stress on my joints. My pantry had to contain only small packaged items that were easy for me to lift and use. My cooking utensils required large handles that are easy to hold and maneuver.

The day-to-day necessities and operational requirements of life had to be on the main floor of our home for easy access. Realizing that my laundry room was downstairs and bedroom upstairs, I needed to limit my use of the stairs as much as possible. I had to organize Samantha's bedroom so she had access to everything herself and became self-sufficient versus reliant on me. Lastly, in order to maintain a clean and orderly home, I needed to hire a cleaning service since I could not bend, lift a vacuum or wash floors.

Being a good manager of my illness means working with others to accomplish the day-to-day functions of life. You need to understand the repetitive functions in your life and then learn, practice and master a set of skills that allow for comfortable living.

With the move now complete and Samantha re-established, I needed to focus on looking after me. That meant slowing down my life and managing my stress. If I could accomplish these two things I would be able to reduce the inflammation in my joints that was causing this incredible pain. I also needed to find an exercise program I could take part in to keep my joints from seizing up and I had to pay more attention to my diet. A proper diet prevents undue stress on weight bearing joints and helps maintain an ideal body weight. I had become far too thin and needed to gain back some weight.

A few weeks into my new job I received a call from Cathy Miller. The province of Alberta was in need of a patient-based advocacy group to work with The Arthritis Society and the provincial government to highlight and bring resolution to arthritis related issues. These issues included: the rheumatologist shortage; approval of arthritis medications; education; patient services; and, public awareness. Cathy offered me the opportunity to help create and Chair a grassroots advocacy group within Alberta. Without hesitation, I accepted her offer since it would provide me the chance to learn more about my RA and the challenges facing others suffering from arthritis.

The following year was more than a fresh start for Samantha and me. I took this time to recreate a life for me that would include my illness. I completed the grieving process over a lost life and all its expectations and I reinvented a new life for myself, one that would carry me into the future. The Arthritis Society offers an Arthritis Self-Management Program that is better known as ASMP. This program is designed to help you and your family members understand your arthritis. It teaches you strategies in coping with chronic pain and educates you on how to take a more active role in managing your illness. This program could not have come along at a better time for me and it made a huge difference in helping me cope and manage my illness.

At this time, I also made a number of visits to a clinic in Calgary called Maximum Potential. This clinic specializes in arthritis and its philosophy is to assess accurately, treat appropriately and achieve maximum potential for its patients in their personal and occupational endeavors. With my severe joint pain, I could not find an exercise program that would improve my fitness level and keep my joints mobile. Maximum Potential was able to design a program for me that included range-of-motion exercises and strengthening my joints in addition to paraffin wax treatments that soothed the severe and sharp joint pain I was suffering.

I learned through Maximum Potential it is important to use your joints and muscles efficiently in order to reduce stress, pain and fatigue. When your joints are in good alignment there is less pressure on them and your body is better able to absorb shock. Understanding and paying attention to the principles of body mechanics was an important lesson for me. When you are in pain, learning the proper way to stand, bend and pick up a dropped item makes life's tasks easier to manage.

Also, do not underestimate the impact of good posture. It will help you considerably.

Arthritis and an active life can be difficult to combine when you are experiencing chronic pain, stiffness and fear of further harming yourself. However, a regular exercise program is fundamental to your well being and recovery. A consistent exercise routine should increase your flexibility, strengthen your muscles and joints, give you more stamina, reduce your fatigue and improve your general health and well being.

People suffering from arthritis walk, bike, swim, practice tai chi and yoga as well as engage in many other forms of range-of-motion and strengthening exercises. Professionals say the benefits of regular exercise are endless and most patients report less pain, anxiety and depression.

When others become aware that you have an illness, they can be full of advice. It is important to listen to what they have to say, as there are never too many good ideas. However, use yourself as a resource. This is your illness and no one understands the full effects of your RA better than you. So give the advice some thought but also come up with your own ideas.

If you want information, go to sources such as the internet or the library. You should find the information you need to make sense of what is right for you. I found reading most helpful. I read countless books on RA and how to best manage my illness given the demands of everyday life. Through educating myself about my illness, I was taking back control of my life and shaping my destiny. I was recreating a life for myself that would carry me into the future.

My volunteer work with The Arthritis Society introduced me to a number of quality individuals suffering from this same illness. Speaking with them openly and honestly about their

RA and how it affects them, what works and doesn't work for them and how they are dealing with their illness was invaluable to me. I have had the pleasure of meeting the most wonderful people though the most adverse circumstances. Clearly, I was no longer alone in this fight. I had built a network of friends and professionals who understood my illness and how it affects me. I consider myself fortunate to have a circle of friends I can count on to be loyal, compassionate and understanding no matter how I am feeling and how I am coping with my illness.

For me, this year was more than a typical transition year that most newly separated people experience. For me, this year was one of acceptance, knowledge and growth. Arthritis, like so many other illnesses, is chronic and needs to be managed because cures are usually not possible. I have come to learn that your quality of life and the extent to which your illness affects you are very much up to you.

Acceptance is key and learning to manage your arthritis is the difference between a poor and good quality of life. If you want quality of life for you and those close to you, my advice is invest in yourself because you are worth it and you owe it to yourself and those close to you to live well and thrive with RA.

CHAPTER FOUR
Knowledge Is Power

Having overcome some major milestones in my personal life, I also had to accept that I had rheumatoid arthritis (RA) and I needed to create a new life that worked for me. Quite simply, the life I knew before my diagnosis would not carry me into the future. With no cure for RA on the horizon, my future remains uncertain. Therefore, educating myself about this illness has been a critical component of my success. If you are going to beat this illness and thrive while living with RA, knowledge is power and you need to always operate from a position of strength.

Three elements we are going to focus on in this chapter are:

- Understanding your illness and how it affects you
- Learning about medical treatments that can help you
- Building a core group of health professionals

Understanding Your Illness and How It Affects You

In order to best manage your arthritis it is essential that you accept responsibility for the elements of your illness that are within your control. Acceptance is a key milestone. It will allow you to progress beyond your current state and re-create a more fulfilling life.

Understanding what triggers your RA to flare up is critical to managing the multitude of symptoms and various elements of your illness. Once you understand how your body reacts to your RA, the better equipped you are to manage your illness and achieve better quality of life. Triggers are different for everyone so you need to understand how your RA affects you. Pay careful attention to what your body is telling you and understand the warning signals well in advance of a flare up.

Medical Treatment

As discussed in Chapter Two, the best way to manage the progression of your RA and control your illness is through medication. However, RA is a chronic illness and we also know you will require many forms of medical treatment throughout your diagnosis. You will need to do some research and learn everything you can about the medications you are taking and how they may or may not affect you.

You need to understand what medications are available in the marketplace and which ones can help you achieve wellness. You also need to be aware of new medications that are being studied and developed for future use. As discussed in Chapter One, even though the federal government approves new medications for use, it does not mean people suffering from RA across the country will have access to them. Adding a new medication to the provincial formulary could take anywhere from one to four years. You need to do your homework in order to understand what new medical treatments will be available to you and within what timeframe.

In addition, get in touch with The Arthritis Society and the medical community to learn about what provincial and national research initiatives are underway when it comes to finding a cure for RA. Remember knowledge is power!

Building a Core Group of Health Professionals

The key to achieving wellness is finding a core group of experienced and dedicated health professionals ready to assist you in your quest to improve your quality of life.

Investigate what type of health professionals you require to best manage your illness. Then bring this group together, communicate what is important to you, develop an action plan, measure your progress and deliver the results to all involved to ensure you succeed in your quest to live well.

On days when you are in so much pain and have nothing left to give yourself or anyone else this may seem like a huge challenge. It is at these times that I urge you to dig deep and find the courage and strength to get the job done.

During these difficult times it is critical to remember that failure is not an option. Do not, under any circumstances, surrender to this illness. Now is the time to work with your core group of health professionals and take command of your RA. Your long-term quality of life is at stake and you owe it to yourself and those close to you to do everything possible to win this battle. Maintaining your quality of life is essential.

In order successfully lead your core group of health professionals you need to implement a plan that includes the following steps:

1. Develop strategies based on information gathered from your core group of health professionals.
2. Turn the information into action plan with achievable goals and objectives.
3. Work your plan. Ensure your decisions are being carried out.
4. Measure your plan for progress.
5. Assess and modify your plan to achieve your desired outcome.

Whether you are a natural born leader or not, following these five straight-forward steps will allow you to develop a simple and effective process that will assist you in managing your RA.

There are many types of health care professionals who can assist you in achieving wellness. Your core group should include:

- family doctor
- rheumatologist
- orthopedic surgeon
- nurse
- psychologist
- occupational therapist
- physiotherapist
- massage therapist
- nutritionist
- pharmacist

As a person with a chronic illness you will spend a lot of time with health professionals. Getting the most from your core group of health professionals is essential to improving your quality of life.

Family Doctor

Doctors play a meaningful role in every individual's life. For someone suffering from RA that role is crucial. Your family doctor should be able to answer fundamental questions about arthritis and refer you to a specialist.

Rheumatologist

Rheumatologists are specialists with training in the diagnosis and treatment of arthritis. They are aware of the development of leading-edge drugs and medical treatments and, as a result, provide enormous value to their patients. One of the primary benefits of visiting a rheumatologist is their ability to endorse patients for clinical trials.

Finding the right rheumatologist for you is key to your overall success and since arthritis is a chronic illness it is important to develop an open and comfortable relationship.

This type of relationship does not always occur with the initial referral from your family doctor. Personally, I was first referred to a very competent rheumatologist but he lacked the necessary communication skills needed to discuss my illness and work with me to develop an action plan to improve my quality of life.

As a result, I made the decision to exchange this health professional for someone with better communication skills. My rheumatologist is named Dr. Christopher Penney and he has been my rheumatologist for more than seven years. He is an outstanding doctor and person, is highly regarded by his peers and well recognized in his field. He is extremely knowledgeable and leads the field in a number of rheumatology initiatives. Dr. Penney understands the affects a chronic illness has on his patients and possesses the necessary strength of character to meet his patients needs. I feel blessed to have him working on my behalf. If you are not 100 per cent comfortable, happy or confident with one of your health professionals than I recommend you make change. Your quality of life is too important to trust to someone who cannot deliver what you need.

Orthopedic Surgeon

Should pain, serious joint damage and/or deformity cause you to require an operation to replace joints you will likely involve an orthopedic surgeon as one of your health professionals. Orthopedic surgeons are trained to perform surgery on joints, bones, tendons, and ligaments.

I have been fortunate and, so far, I have not required surgery on my joints. As a result, I do not have an orthopedic surgeon in my core group of health professionals. Should you find yourself looking for this type of health professional, I recommend you contact The Arthritis Society division nearest to you and ask for a list of local practicing orthopedic surgeons. Prior to selecting your orthopedic surgeon you should check their references by speaking to a few of their patients then meet with a selected few who come highly recommended.

Nurse

While doctors are busy visiting patients, nurses are busy organizing the doctors, providing them patient information and caring for their patients. A nurse will provide you with access to both informal and formal professional help, advice and information. In addition to administering medications by intravenous or injection when required. Having a nurse in your core group of health professionals is invaluable.

Psychologist

Acceptance and coming to terms with your RA is a key milestone to moving forward and re-creating a life that will carry you into the future. If you are challenged or having problems working through the physical and emotional impacts of RA I recommend you seek professional assistance. Looking back, this is a service I should have taken advantage of but did not. Seeking professional assistance would have helped me come to terms with my RA earlier and improved my quality of life much sooner.

Occupational Therapist (OT)

Occupational Therapists teach you how to handle the demands of everyday life with a chronic illness. They teach you how to get things done with minimum pain, stress and fatigue. Having an OT in your core group of health professionals provides you with coping strategies that are essential to managing your illness and maintaining your independence.

In the early days of being diagnosed with RA, my rheumatologist sent me to the Rockyview Hospital in Calgary for an assessment. My hands and wrists were so sore I could barely move them. The OT taught me how to hold my blow dryer with minimal pain so I could dry my hair. Since the joints in my fingers and hands were inflamed and swollen I could not pick up small items. As a result, the OT exposed me to a line of kitchen utensils called Handy Grips. These kitchen utensils are designed for people suffering from RA because they have big handles, are lightweight and easy to use. As a young mother, my biggest challenge was learning how to properly lift and balance my daughter Samantha, her diaper bag and my purse. The OT taught me to balance all this with less joint pressure and pain. Learning these techniques made the demands of everyday life much easier to cope with.

Physiotherapist (PT)

When it comes to range-of-motion your PT will provide you with a physical examination and assessment for all your major joints. The PT will then develop a physiotherapy plan consisting of two to four, forty-five minute treatments per week that will include range-of-motion and strengthening exercises to help keep you flexible and mobile.

If you live in Calgary, there is no better organization to assist you in the area of mobility than Maximum Potential. This organization has trained PTs you can add to your core group of health professionals with a great deal of experience in meeting the needs of arthritis patients. My PT assessed my range-of-motion and developed a program with a series of exercises for me to complete both on-site or off. I would highly recommend this organization to anyone suffering from any form of arthritis.

Massage Therapist (MT)

When it comes to RA massage is the simplest form of physical treatment and it can alleviate pain. If you are considering adding a MT to your core group of health professionals seek a licensed practitioner with experience in treating people with RA.

Personally, massage therapy was not a treatment I could benefit from when I was in severe pain. If my pain was moderate and manageable only then could I receive value from this form of treatment. Massage therapy is one of the easiest and more affordable ways to increase your overall well being. I get massages monthly now that my RA is in remission.

Nutritionist

As part of your core group of health professionals a nutritionist can prove worthwhile. For example, do you know how foods interact with your medication? Some forms of arthritis can be triggered by food. Therefore, understanding what foods are known to worsen or improve RA symptoms is extremely valuable.

When you are healthy it is easy to devalue the role of a nutritionist and well-balanced diet. Only after I was diagnosed with RA did I focus on eating properly and maintaining a healthy diet. This change in lifestyle allowed me to maintain an appropriate body weight, possess the energy I needed to get through the day and prevent undue stress on weight-bearing joints. This is an element of your treatment that you have control over and should pay proper attention to.

Pharmacist

When it comes to selecting a pharmacist to join your core group of health professionals it is important to choose someone you feel comfortable with and trust. If you have questions regarding how to take your medication or a reaction to it and cannot see your specialist right away, your pharmacist can be very helpful.

I have had only two pharmacists during my illness. The first one was excellent but retired five years into my illness.

The second pharmacist is just as good, if not better. He reviews the medications I am taking and advises me on how and when to take them to avoid a reaction. My pharmacist understands that when I am in pain I do not want gaining access to my medication to be a chore and he has it delivered to me. A pharmacist you like, feel comfortable with and trust is an important member of your core group of health professionals.

Alternative Remedies

Alternative remedies are becoming more popular for people suffering from RA. Prior to any use of alternative remedies you should consult your family doctor or rheumatologist to ensure there is no conflict with current medications you may be taking.

As leader of your core group of health professionals, your active participation and direction are important to achieving your desired outcome. Begin by being prepared for your appointments. If you are seeing a specialist, have your family doctor forward copies of your medical records and X-rays to your specialist prior to your visit. Specialists are very busy and you will probably spend some time on a waiting list before you see one, so be prepared. Write down any questions you may have and prioritize them. Should your appointment be cut short or you run out of time it is essential to get your most important questions answered. If it is a repeat visit, prepare a report of what has transpired since your last appointment and be ready to discuss it in detail. Inform your specialist of your goals and objectives with in addition to other members of your core group of health professionals. The more information each of them has about the other and your experiences, the more pertinent and informed their recommendations will be.

It is important to explore all forms of treatment options with your core group of health professionals. Before accepting any form of treatment you should do your research and educate yourself on the pros and cons of the recommended treatment. If you are unsure or object to the recommended treatment based on your experience with your illness, get a second opinion. If the same treatment is prescribed, work to find a mutually acceptable solution or alternative.

Communicating your goals and objectives to your core group of health professionals is essential. It is important to communicate and share this information with those close to you as they are your support network and in a position to help you improve your quality of life. In addition, you need to accept responsibility for elements of your illness that are within your control. A healthy lifestyle is crucial to your success as it can greatly influence the results of your treatment. It is vital to exercise regularly, eat well, get the proper amount of rest and stay active. A healthy lifestyle will help you maintain a positive attitude and outlook on life, a key to managing your illness and winning this battle.

In summary, knowledge is power and you always want to be operating from a position of strength. To accomplish this you need to understand your illness and how it affects you, learn about medical treatments that can help you and develop a core group of health professionals committed to achieving your desired outcome, thriving with rheumatoid arthritis

CHAPTER FIVE
Pain Management

Controlling pain is the number one issue for people suffering from rheumatoid arthritis (RA). Each person's experience with arthritis pain is exclusive to them. It usually cannot be seen by others and it is hard to explain, which makes it difficult to comprehend, contend with and control. As discussed in Chapter Two, the best way to control pain is through medication. Having said that, medication does not completely eliminate RA pain so additional insight is required.

RA is a chronic illness. Once diagnosed, it never goes away so recognizing and living your reality is vital to understanding the various elements of pain and managing their effects.

Normal pain is something we feel physically and something we have feelings about emotionally. Pain, especially acute short-term pain, often works as an alarm system telling us to change our activity or environment to stop or lessen the pain. Chronic pain is more challenging because the source of pain cannot be removed.

Pain starts when special receptors are stimulated in the affected area. A pain message is sent along the nerves to the spinal cord, which has special "gate mechanisms" that can either reduce or increase the incoming pain message. The message then travels to the brain's pain center where it is given both physical and emotional meaning.

We all have individual thresholds for pain and those tolerances change from day-to-day, depending on a variety of factors. It is important to remember that pain means different things to different people and not all people experience pain from their arthritis in the same way. That is why what works to relieve pain for one person may not necessarily work for another.

The pain cycle for RA can be related to at least three elements of the illness:

- Physical (increased disease activity, pain, fatigue, disturbed sleep, etc.)
- Emotional (stress, mood, anxiety, depression, etc.)
- Other factors (personality, culture, beliefs, attitude about pain and illness, etc.)

Arthritis may cause you pain due to inflammation of the joints or bone rubbing against bone. In response to this pain, and to protect the area that hurts, your body unconsciously tends to tighten the muscles of the affected area or compensates by using other muscles. When these muscles are tightened for long periods of time, they create even more pain. This is the physical element of your illness. As your pain mounts, you become more stressed and more tense as you question if the pain will ever get better. Your pain may force you to cut back on everyday activities. This in turn may trigger depression, anger, or frustration and make the pain feel even worse. This is the emotional element of your illness. These two elements lead you to the "other factors" element of your illness. This determines whether you have the ability to take charge of your symptoms and maintain your quality of life. These three elements complete the RA pain cycle.

As demonstrated above, RA pain comes from many sources so it is important to recognize what is causing you pain to ensure pain management techniques are aimed at the appropriate sources. It is only once you understand what is your source of pain that you can apply techniques to help control it.

Heat and cold are often used to assist with the physical pain element including inflammation of joints, surrounding tissue, and bone rubbing on bone. They are effective and inexpensive ways to achieve temporary relief. Heat is excellent for relieving muscle tension and stiffness. It works by increasing the blood flow to the skin and muscles around the painful area. When muscles relax, the pain and stiffness decrease. Methods you can use to apply heat include warm baths and showers, a hot tub, sauna, steam room or a heating pad. Paraffin wax treatments can be excellent, depending on the area of discomfort. For some, applying cold works better to stop muscle spasms and numb the nerves that are sending pain signals. Plastic storage bags filled with ice or ice packs work well. When using ice it is important to wrap it in a towel or cloth to avoid skin burn from the cold. Creams and/or liniments applied in addition to massage are also effective.

The lack of, or poor quality of, sleep interferes with our ability to cope with pain and get through the day. In Canada, arthritis affects more than four million people and in other countries a greater population is affected. As a result, mattress manufacturers are producing arthritis friendly mattresses for people with this illness to facilitate a good night's rest. If you are not sleeping well, then I suggest you look into a mattress that works for you, as sleep is a key element to controlling pain. In addition to a proper mattress, sleeping aids are also available.

Fatigue is a common symptom of arthritis sufferers. It can be caused by many things, including:

- active disease
- lack of physical fitness
- depression (fatigue can be a sign of depression)
- poor nutrition
- medications
- stress
- lack of sleep or interrupted sleep

Exercise is an excellent means of overcoming fatigue, especially if it is caused by depression or lack of fitness versus the disease process. Other ways of managing fatigue include scheduling frequent rest periods during the day and alternating heavy and light work during each day. Examining your lifestyle and life philosophy are important to ensure you are setting yourself up for success and not failure. Also, it is vital to be organized, plan ahead and, most importantly, use your joints wisely. Effective fatigue management is an excellent way to help break the pain cycle by rejuvenating both the mind and body.

Controlling the physical pain is not the only symptom of RA; other symptoms are centered on the emotional element of this illness. When first diagnosed with arthritis, patients experience a myriad of emotions. Shock, disbelief and denial are common thoughts. Fear and panic surface next as life is quickly changing, you are unable to keep up and you are becoming more dependent on others for everyday tasks. As time progresses there is uncertainty and frustration over how one day you can live an almost normal life and the next day you are not able to function. Anger is a common emotion aimed at the unfairness of the illness along with feelings of "why me?" Depression and sadness over a lost life and shattered dreams are emotions shared by most everyone suffering from this illness.

Depression is a frequent problem for chronic pain sufferers.

Like pain and fatigue, depression can easily contribute to an increasing cycle of pain. Recognizing depression is the first step to overcoming it. How do you know if you are depressed? A person may experience any one or any combination of the following symptoms:

- loss of interest in friends or activities
- isolation or withdrawal
- difficulty or changes in sleep patterns
- increased or decreased appetite
- loss of interest in personal care or appearance
- unintentional weight loss or gain
- general feeling of unhappiness, crying
- loss of interest in sex, intimacy
- suicidal thoughts
- frequent accidents
- low self-image, loss of self-esteem
- frequent arguments or loss of temper
- feeling tired or fatigued
- feeling confused, lack of concentration

To overcome depression it is important to keep in contact with others, plan ahead for special events, get out of the house everyday, do something nice for yourself, engage in some kind of exercise (like walking or stretching) or do something to help someone else. It is important to be aware that not all depression can be handled through self-management. Severe depression requires professional help and medication. If you feel unhappy for more than a few weeks, or think about harming yourself, it is important to talk to your doctor. Severe clinical depression is a biological illness and can be treated.

While we can't eliminate stress from our lives, there are many ways to minimize its impact. Relaxation exercises are a common form of reducing stress levels in today's busy environment. Meditation and imagery exercises are available on cassette tape or CD at your local library or for purchase at your bookstore.

To properly manage the emotional element of your illness you need to accept that you have RA. You need to take charge of the symptoms and elements of the illness within your control even if you are unsure of what your future may look like. Acceptance is a key milestone. It will allow you to progress beyond your current state and re-create a life that will carry you into the future.

When it comes to controlling pain and your emotional well being it is important to put aside any stereotypes, whether cultural or preconceived beliefs about pain and illness. No personal or social belief should stand in the way of you beating this illness and improving your quality of life. I am a big believer in attitude, and with the right attitude I believe you can thrive with rheumatoid arthritis.

Understanding what triggers your RA is critical to managing the various symptoms and elements of your illness. Once you understand how your body reacts to your RA, the better equipped you are to control the physical pain and deal with the emotional symptoms that are keeping you from achieving good quality of life. Triggers are different for everyone and no two arthritis sufferers are the same. For some people it is food related, for others it is stress related.

Throughout my illness my triggers have remained constant. Stress and lack of sleep have the ability to send me into a flare up and render me bedridden. With the demands of raising Samantha, running a household and managing my career I have to pay careful attention to what my body is saying and understand the warning signals.

Prior to Remicade, there were times I was in so much pain

that at the end of the day I had nothing left to give anyone else. I was physically, emotionally and mentally exhausted. More often than not I found myself living in a cocoon of pain, immobile and unable to care for myself. I was not living the life I had envisioned for myself. I merely existed through each passing day.

To maintain some form of normalcy and not allow your pain to consume you it is essential that you manage your RA triggers. You also need to keep active when you are in pain and not give in and stay in bed. It is important to get up, shower, dress and go to work. If you don't work, go somewhere else, visit a friend. Do not sit at home and become a martyr to this illness.

Throughout my journey with RA I have learned that pain is individual. It can not be seen so don't be afraid to let those close to you know you are in pain and need help. Always ask for help when required, a direct ask for assistance is not being dependent. It is open, honest and necessary communication.

Arthritis is a chronic illness and as a result you live with anxiety and uncertainty. This illness causes you to experience a series of physical and emotional highs and lows. One day you live an almost normal life and the next day you are immobile. Throughout this illness it is important to let those close to you know what you are dealing with so you can set limitations and reasonable expectations of what you are capable of.

Whether you are suffering with the physical pain of this illness or its emotional effects, is important to accept, understand and work to overcome these elements of your illness. In times like these you need to be honest with yourself, decide what is important to you and then look for ways to achieve your goals. Don't worry about how you get there, whether you do it alone or with help. Just focus on your outcome.

There is no doubt suffering with RA as a young person, or at any age, is a challenge. However, I believe that your quality of life and how you are impacted by your illness are very much up to you. With the right attitude, you can lead a fulfilling life and thrive with rheumatoid arthritis.

CHAPTER SIX
Becoming An Arthritis Advocate

Becoming an arthritis advocate was never part of my plan, even after I was first diagnosed with rheumatoid arthritis (RA). Five years into my illness it became apparent there were three fundamental areas of my life that would always be impacted by my illness. These three areas were:

- my personal well being and health,
- my relationship with my daughter Samantha, and
- the public's lack of understanding regarding my illness.

The entire concept that "arthritis is an old person's disease" is one that must be changed.

These three components of my life were becoming a re-occurring theme and resonated with me in a very meaningful and sincere way. They have compelled me to advocate on behalf of myself, my daughter and others suffering from arthritis.

When it comes to personal well being and health, I am pleased with how I have come to terms with my arthritis. This was a life-altering experience for me. Understanding and accepting my illness has allowed me to move beyond my pain and physical limitations. I have re-created a well-balanced life for me and my daughter that is fun and fulfilling. With no cure for arthritis in sight I also know that my journey has not come to an end and I may be required to travel down that hard, painful road once again. However, I know now that if need be

I can travel that road confident in the knowledge that I can manage my personal quality of life and my daughter's future.

As Samantha would say, "My mom does a lot of different things." Of all the things I do, mothering Samantha and helping her develop into a successful young woman is the most important. I believe it is essential to be a good role model for your children and lead by example. As Samantha would also say, "walk your talk." As for my RA and how it has affected my family, the message I want to send Samantha is that it is not about what happens to you in life, it is how you choose to deal with it that matters. Adversity is really about having the strength of character to step up, face your fears, and ascertain your desired outcome. When your health and family are in jeopardy, failure is not an option!

I believe the best way to generate public awareness for arthritis is to have the people who have been diagnosed with this crippling and debilitating illness, or people close to them, tell their stories. It is the real life stories of arthritis sufferers, as well as spouses, children and parents, which touch the general public and raise their level of awareness, understanding and knowledge. Watching someone you know and care about struggle to maintain their quality of life and everything that is "normal" to them is an eye-opener. I believe by generating public awareness for people suffering from RA will call attention to the issues and help bring about timely and proper medical treatment.

My diagnosis with RA prompted me to contact The Arthritis Society in Calgary. My experience with this organization and the people employed or volunteering within it both provincially and nationally has been first rate. The Arthritis Society invests its time in improving the lives of the four million Canadians suffering from arthritis. It provides a variety of treatment and education programs, lobby's governments on health-care policy and invests in research and development to find a cure. The Arthritis Society improves the quality of life for people suffering from arthritis. Although at first hesitant about contacting The Arthritis Society, getting involved and building relationships both provincially and nationally has given me an opportunity to contribute to a select group of people I have something in common. It has also enriched my life with the most wonderful friendships.

Through my involvement with this organization I have learned a lot about my illness and how to manage it. I have also learned a lot about the challenges facing the organization. Once I developed an understanding of the challenges both provincially and nationally I felt compelled to roll up my sleeves and work as a volunteer with the staff of The Arthritis Society to make change.

In the Alberta and Northwest Territories Division I was privileged to work with Cathy Miller, Beth Kidd and other senior staff to implement a grass-roots advocacy group called the Arthritis Consumers Team (ACT) for the province in 1998. Working closely with Beth, we established four key areas that needed a profile and recruited a dozen volunteers with and without arthritis to assist us in these areas.

A Speakers Bureau was formed to generate both public and consumer (or patient) awareness. We polled our volunteers and worked with a few who had an interest in this area to develop a plan to recruit speakers and train them on arthritis issues so they could then educate the public and generate broader awareness of the disease. It is important that The Arthritis Society maintain a current volunteer speaker's directory for future public relations and media events.

A Member Assistance Group was created to provide

services to people suffering from arthritis. Action plans were developed and implemented to research and initiate a family/partner support group and a peer-support group (or buddy system) for people newly diagnosed with arthritis. This group of volunteers was also responsible for improving the provincial arthritis telephone help line.

A Health Professional Group was formed to deal with arthritis patients and doctors. Volunteers with an interest in this area developed and implemented action plans to educate general practitioners on arthritis so they could refer their patients to the appropriate specialist. In addition, a patient brochure was developed for people newly diagnosed with arthritis. It contained relevant questions to ask both their general practitioner and any specialist. This group also investigated methods to improve the compassionate drug programs offered by the pharmaceutical companies.

A Government Relations Group was created to inform provincial government officials and other key decision makers on arthritis issues and concerns. In addition to Chairing ACT, government relations was my passion so I also decided to get involved and became Chair of this group. Together with some dedicated volunteers we developed and implemented action plans to ensure patients had access to new medications and we produced a list of tax relief benefits available to people with arthritis. We also supported the roll-out of The Arthritis Society's Canadian Arthritis Bill of Rights and developed short-term and long-term objectives to deal with the shortage of rheumatologists in Alberta. In addition, we circulated a quarterly newsletter outlining arthritis issues and concerns to about thirty key decision makers in the provincial and federal governments. We also met with the Alberta Minister of Health and Wellness three times per year to enhance the arthritis profile.

Working with The Arthritis Society's Alberta Division and a group of outstanding volunteers, ACT was able to achieve its goals and objectives in the province and generate national news. To have the opportunity to be there at the start, build and lead this exceptional group of people for the following two years was an honor. As Chair of ACT, Cathy and Beth requested I give a presentation on arthritis issues to Arthritis Rheumatism International. This organization was hosting a conference in Edmonton called Action Against Arthritis, Taking Charge in the 21st Century. This was my first formal presentation on behalf of The Arthritis Society and it was to an audience of approximately two hundred and fifty people either diagnosed with arthritis, affected by arthritis or health professionals.

Shortly after, Denis Morrice, the Chief Executive Officer and President of The Arthritis Society in Canada asked me if I would sit on a Steering Committee with eight other volunteers to launch a national grass-roots advocacy group called the Canadian Arthritis Patient Alliance (CAPA). Again, another outstanding opportunity was presented to me. I had to think about this since I had a career, a daughter to raise, five to ten hours a week of volunteer work with ACT and, don't forget, I have RA so looking after me was a priority. After some discussion with Denis about the time commitment to CAPA, I said yes and was off to Toronto for my first meeting on how to bring this group together.

My participation in CAPA at the national level was really interesting. I met people from all over Canada who had some form of arthritis and, to my surprise, the issues were not much different than what ACT was working to change in Alberta. My confidence was high because ACT was already achieving what this group wanted to develop and implement.

I immediately knew I found my niche and my experience with ACT would really make a difference.

I was pumped and I proposed a divisional model to the group. A divisional model would allow the people from across the country at the table to create synergy, share information and learning's in the provinces and nationally. There was no need to reinvent the wheel. All we needed to do was take what we knew worked and build on it. When it came time to fly back to Calgary after the weekend I was pleased with the progress we had made and was looking forward to our next meeting in two months.

Back at home things were running smoothly with ACT and it was time to start the succession planning process for me and other key individuals. I believe new blood is imperative to the success of any organization and after a year and a half we needed to refresh and I needed to move on. During the transition of our incoming Chair I stayed on as Government Relations Chair for an extra six months to provide continuity and support. My passion is building, so I knew I would want to move on to another challenge soon.

Shortly after returning home, I was invited to travel to Slovenia with five other volunteers to represent The Arthritis Society of Canada at a worldwide conference called International League of Arthritis Rheumatism. I consulted with my employer, Colt Engineering, as to whether the timing was appropriate for me to go. Colt aware of my involvement with The Arthritis Society was once again very supportive and sent me on my way. This conference proved to be one more great opportunity in the many I have had with The Arthritis Society. It was an honor to be chosen to attend and represent The Arthritis Society of Canada and I enjoyed participating in the discussions at the conference.

Upon my return, my next challenge awaited me. The timing could not have been better as biologic drugs designed for arthritis sufferers were new to Canada and Canadians could not access them. These new drugs were something I understood and could relate to since a few months earlier I was invited to join a "trial program" put on by Schering Canada, officially known as a special access program, for a new biologic called Remicade. These programs are designed to demonstrate the patient benefits of new innovations and speed up the approval process for the pharmaceutical companies seeking to distribute their drugs.

While I only had two infusions, clearly Remicade was a wonder drug and my arthritis was quickly becoming more manageable. I also met a number of people in Slovenia who had access to these drugs for some time and they were receiving tremendous benefit from them. A new challenge fell right in my lap at the right time. As Chair of the Government Relations Group in Alberta, Beth and I developed federal and provincial strategies to ensure arthritis patients could gain access to both Remicade and the competing drug Enbrel. This plan also included the national office of The Arthritis Society and CAPA. It was an excellent opportunity to leverage the expertise and passion both staff and volunteers brought to the table.

To the surprise of most patients in both the Remicade and Enbrel trial programs, we learned that each province must apply separately to have these biologic drugs added to their formularies. The Government of Canada approved Remicade and Enbrel three months into our fight, but that did not mean all of the people suffering from RA across the country would have access to them. As a group of patients now experiencing a quality of life we had long hoped for, we were concerned about our future. With more than 400,000 people with arthritis in Alberta, we assumed Alberta would be one of the first provinces to grant access to these new biologics. To our dismay, Alberta was one of the last provinces to add these drugs to its formulary. This left patients like me wondering if we would receive our medication at all or if we would have to pay for it ourselves. This was maddening, not to mention unethical.

There were about two hundred and thirty Albertans on this trial program and all were candidates for either short-term or long-term disability if they didn't receive their medication. For the first time since our diagnosis of RA, a large number of us were in good health and enjoying better quality of life. If you took a close look at these statistics and built an economic model based upon them it was clear that the cost of approving these drugs in all the provinces, especially Alberta, was nominal and paid for itself in short order. Which begged the question, if it made sense then why hadn't the Government of Alberta approved these drugs for funding?

It quickly became obvious that people suffering from arthritis needed to make more noise. So we did. I was happy to lead this effort in Alberta and it resulted in both Remicade and Enbrel finally being approved and added to the provincial formulary. With this task complete, I retired as Chair of the Government Relations Group and accepted a position on the Division Board of Directors as a Director at Large.

Sitting on the Alberta and Northwest Territories Board of Directors provided me with a clear understanding of how The Arthritis Society functions. It is a governance Board meaning we set the vision and direction and leave Cathy and her staff to handle the day-to-day operations in executing our vision. This was a little different than what I was used to. Typically in my other roles, I made things happen. Sitting on this Board was going to develop my leadership skills and I was excited about that. After my first year as a Director at Large I was appointed Vice-Chair, which meant I was being fast-tracked to become the Chair.

My role as Chair began in June 2003 with a two-year commitment through to June 2005 following another two-year commitment as Past Chair ending in June 2007. Our mission is to improve the quality of life for people affected with arthritis and to support proactive efforts directed toward prevention, diagnosis, treatment and a cure for arthritis.

In my first year as Chair of the Alberta and Northwest Territories Board, I was invited to join the National Board of Directors as a Director at Large. I accepted, attended my first meeting in June 2004 and I look forward to contributing in a meaningful way to a select group of people whom I admire and share a common interest in improving the quality of life for those suffering with arthritis.

As I mentioned at the start of this chapter, becoming an arthritis advocate was never part of my game plan. However, since then I have been honored for my service with many awards including:

- The Arthritis Society Outstanding Volunteer Award
- The Arthritis Hero Award of Recognition
- The Queen's 50th Anniversary Golden Jubilee Medal

When you contribute your time and effort to a cause you truly believe in awards and medals are never an expectation. Having said that, I am genuinely humbled and appreciative of these honors.

My volunteer service with The Arthritis Society has introduced me to a number of extraordinary people suffering from RA and other forms of arthritis. Speaking with them honestly about how their arthritis affects them, what treatments work and don't work for them and how they are dealing with their illness continues to be invaluable to me. Throughout my involvement with this organization I have had the pleasure of meeting the most amazing and courageous people though the most adverse circumstances.

Clearly, I am no longer alone in my fight to conquer my RA and through giving back I have built a network of health professionals who are essential for me to achieve wellness and improve my quality of life throughout my struggles with RA. I have also developed some wonderful new friends who I can add to my existing circle of cherished friendships. There is not a day that goes by that I don't feel privileged to have been given the opportunity to become a part of The Arthritis Society and contribute to such an exceptional organization and group of people.

Twelve years into this illness, I have surpassed some major milestones. I have come to accept that I have this terrible illness and I have created a new life that works for me. I feel I have acquired the strength of character to step up, face my fears and ascertain my desired outcome and I believe you can too. My advice to you throughout your journey with RA is to "fight" and "fight hard." Your quality of life and the lives of those close to you depend on your success when it comes to managing your illness. No matter what the circumstance, failure is not an option and you too can thrive with rheumatoid arthritis.

REFERENCE MATERIAL

Conquering Rheumatoid Arthritis

Authors: William Bensen, M.D.

Wynn Bensen, BA

Control Pain Management Workshop

Authors: The Arthritis Society

Alberta & N.W.T Division

The Arthritis Society Website

www.arthritis.ca

About the Author

By day, Linda is a Sales & Marketing Executive. By night Linda advocates on behalf of people suffering from arthritis.

Linda resides on The Arthritis Society's Divisional and National Board of Directors and the Scientific Advisory Committee.

Linda has been honored with many awards for her contribution. A few are noted below:

- Outstanding Volunteer Award;

- Arthritis Hero Award of Recognition; and

- The Queen's Fifth Anniversary Golden Jubilee Medal.